I0696275

TABLE OF CONTENT

Chapter 1: Understanding Fertility

1.1 The Miracle of Conception

Having a baby may seem simple, but the reality of conception and pregnancy is far from simple. On the contrary, it is actually extremely complicated. There are many stages in the process where the chain of events may break down. It's no surprise that some people experience problems with getting pregnant. In any given month, couples age 28-33 with normal functioning reproductive systems have only a 20-25 per cent chance of conceiving. After six months of trying, only 60% of couples will conceive without medical assistance.

Most of the time, a woman won't know the exact day she conceived or got pregnant. She may count the start of pregnancy from the first day of the last period. Normally, an egg lives for about 12-24 hours after it's released. For you to get pregnant, a sperm must fertilize the egg within this time. Sperm can live for up to five days inside the woman's body. This means, if the couple have sex up to seven days before the woman ovulates, or within a day or so of ovulating, she could conceive.

It can be inferred that intercourse few days before ovulation can lead to conception. As long as one sperm remains alive, there is a chance of conception. About 24 hours after ovulation, the risk of pregnancy disappears when the woman's egg dies.

The steps to conception and pregnancy are quite complex and it's a miracle that it happens at all. First, the couple must have intercourse every other day around the time of ovulation, because sperm live for an average of 48 hours. Not only must the woman ovulate a mature egg, it must be picked up by a healthy Fallopian Tube; the man must produce sufficient healthy and strongly swimming sperm; the sperm must reach the egg; the egg must change its structure to become a fertilized embryo; genetic material of the embryo must be correct; the embryo must divide correctly to form a blastocyst; and the blastocyst must implant in the womb and be accepted. The wall of the womb must be healthy and ready to allow a fertilized embryo to implant.

This is only just the beginning. Failure of the sperm or egg to make an important connection anywhere along this complicated itinerary will prevent pregnancy from occurring. And to complicate matters, genetic miscoding will often lead to the embryo not implanting, or disintegrating soon after implantation. At this moment of implantation, pregnancy has officially occurred and the placental tissue begins to secrete a hormone called hCG. Implantation may take place as early as a handful of days after ovulation or well over a week. On average, one can expect implantation to occur about six to twelve days after ovulation.

It is estimated that 60- 80 per cent of all naturally conceived embryos are simply flushed out in women's normal menstrual flows unnoticed. And the older a woman gets, the less chance she has of getting pregnant. Women aged

40 and above have only a 5% chance or less of becoming pregnant naturally in any one month.

The process of conception begins quite simply, and then gets really complicated. Every month, the female ovulates one mature egg from one of her ovaries. This egg leaves the ovarian follicle and is 'captured' in the end of the Fallopian tube. Here, it will begin to move slowly down the tube towards the womb (uterus). However, for a pregnancy to develop, it must first meet sperm from the male at the same time as it is still held in the Fallopian tube.

So, how does the sperm get to the egg? Good question. A man ejaculates an average quantity of semen, containing between 100 million and 300 million sperm. Less than 100,000 of them manage to pass through the cervix (opening of the womb). Only about 200 will make it through the Fallopian tubes and only one will fertilize the egg.

The sperm leave the man's penis by ejaculation and are deposited in the vagina high up near the cervix. The sperm immediately begin swimming and some will find their way into the cervix. Sperms have a long journey towards the egg. From the cervix they enter the womb and swim towards the Fallopian tubes. Strangely, the vagina and the womb are not very friendly environments for sperm, but once inside the Fallopian tubes, the ejaculated sperm find their way to the egg. Once they meet, the process of fertilization begins. Many sperm will bind to the shell of the egg, but only one sperm will be allowed to go all the way through to reach the egg inside the shell.

Sperm can survive for a few days in the female reproductive system. Once the sperm has gained entry to the egg, a complex chain of events occurs over a period of about 16-24 hours. Following this, the egg can now be said to be a fertilized embryo and would normally be at this stage one day after ovulation.

For the next few days, the embryo's genetic material divides and then enters the blastocyst stage. From the Fallopian tube, the blastocyst enters the womb. Over the next few days, it hatches out of its shell and attaches or implants into the wall of the womb. It will grow and eventually form blood vessel connections with the mother. This stage of connecting with the womb wall is called "implantation" and is another critical stage in achieving a pregnancy.

At this point, a pregnancy test would be positive. The embryo continues to grow and develop the different types of cells and structures necessary to become a baby. The process of conception has occurred and the woman can now be said to be pregnant.

1.2 The Anatomy of Fertility

The reproductive organs make up an intricate system within a woman's body. The uterus, also called the womb, grows a special lining (endometrium) each month that is shed during a woman's menstrual period. If fertilization and embryo implantation occur, the lining helps to nurture the developing baby. The uterus expands in size as the baby grows.

Most women have two ovaries, which are on either side of the uterus. Eggs are stored in a woman's ovaries. Typically, one egg is released by one ovary each month in a process called ovulation. Ovaries also produce different amounts of hormones, including estrogen, testosterone and progesterone, at different times of the monthly cycle. The fallopian tubes extend from the uterus to each ovary and serve as a passageway for the sperm to reach the egg and afterward for a fertilized embryo to travel to the uterus.

The cervix, found at the base of the uterus, secretes mucus, the consistency of which varies with the stages in the menstrual cycle. At ovulation, cervical mucus is clear, runny and conducive to facilitating the movement of sperm. Post-ovulation, the mucus becomes thicker and more difficult for sperm to swim through. When a pregnant woman is ready to deliver her baby, the cervix dilates, or widens, to allow the baby to pass through the vaginal canal. The entrance to the vagina is located in a woman's vulva, which includes other parts of external genitalia such as the labia, clitoris and urethra. The vulva has two sets of skin folds, or lips. The thinner, inner folds are known as the labia minora, and the thicker, outer ones are the labia majora. Near the top of the vulva is the clitoris, which is a small structure that is sensitive to sexual stimulation. The opening to the urethra, where urine is released from the body, is also found near the top of the vulva, below the clitoris and above the vaginal opening.

The male reproductive system includes the penis, testicles (testes), the system of ducts known as the epididymis and the vas deferens, and the accessory glands, which generate fluids that nourish sperm and lubricate the ducts.

The penis has three parts: the root, the shaft and the glans (or head). All males are born with a foreskin covering the glans of the penis, which is sometimes removed by circumcision. The tip of the penis has an opening that leads to the urethra. The urethra is the tube that passes through the shaft of the penis and releases urine during urination or semen during ejaculation.

The penis contains cylinders of spongy, erectile tissue. During arousal, these become filled with blood, causing an erection, which is necessary for penetration. Semen, a fluid that contains sperm, is released (ejaculated) when a man reaches sexual climax.

Males produce sperm constantly in the testes (testicles), which are located in the scrotum, a pouch-like structure that hangs behind and/or below the penis. Most men have two testicles, which are also responsible for producing testosterone, a hormone that helps the male reproductive system function.

Normal body temperature is too hot for sperm to survive, which is why the testicles are located outside the body proper and in the scrotum, where the temperature is about 3.6 degrees lower. Sperm moves from the testes to the epididymis, which are coiled tubes (one in each testicle) where sperm are stored and reach maturity.

The male anatomy also includes accessory glands, including the prostate gland, Cowper's glands and the seminal vesicles, which create fluids that nourish sperm and lubricate the epididymis and the vas deferens. The vas deferens is a muscular tube that transports semen from the epididymis into the urethra during ejaculation.

Semen contains sperm along with mucus (to protect the sperm from the acid secreted in the vagina), proteins and fructose (the main energy source for the sperm), and prostaglandins that stimulate female uterine contractions, helping move the semen up into the uterus.

1.3 The Men's Role in Fertility

The role of men in fertility is crucial and it is essential to recognize the significant contribution they make to the process of conception. Fertility, which is the ability to conceive a child, is a responsibility shared between partners. Much of the focus of fertility centers around women but understanding the men's role is also important. Here's the role of men in fertility:

Sperm Production: Starting at puberty, men produce sperm continuously throughout their lives. The microscopic swimmers are essential for fertilizing the female egg and initiate the embryo's development.

Sperm Quality: The health and quality of sperm is essential. Sperm should be present in sufficient numbers, motile and well formed as poor sperm quality could lead to difficulties in fertilization.

Lifestyle Choices: The men's choices on their lifestyles have a direct impact on sperm health.

Excessive alcohol consumption, smoking, recreational drug use and poor dietary habits are factors that can affect the quality of sperm

Environmental Exposures: Exposure to environmental toxins, radiation, and certain workplace hazards can have adverse effects on sperm production and function. It's important for men to be aware of potential risks and take necessary precautions.

Sexual Function: The ability to achieve and maintain erection is essential for conception. Sexual health issues or erectile dysfunction can pose barriers to fertility.

Reproductive Anatomy: Any abnormalities, blockages or infections in the male reproductive system such as testes, the epididymis, the urethra and vas deferens can affect fertility.

Hormone Balance: Sperm regulation is influenced by the hormones. Testosterone, luteinizing hormone (LH), and follicle-stimulating hormone (FSH) are among the hormones that influence male reproductive health. Hormonal imbalances can disrupt sperm production.

Genetic Factors: Klinefelter syndrome or Y chromosome deletions in men are factors or conditions that can lead to infertility.

Sexually Transmitted Infections (STIs): Infections like chlamydia and gonorrhea can cause scarring and blockages in the male reproductive tract, leading to fertility issues.

Age: Male fertility can decline but this is less pronounced in women. Advanced paternal age is related with a higher risk of certain genetic conditions in offspring.

Emotional and Psychological Factors: Sexual functions and fertility can be impacted by mental health and emotional wellbeing. Stress, anxiety, and depression can affect the ability to perform sexually.

Medical Conditions: Certain medical conditions like diabetes, obesity and chronic diseases can affect fertility. One needs to manage these conditions through lifestyle changes and medical treatment.

Regular Sexual Activity: Regular and accurately timed sexual activity is essential to optimize fertility. Both the timing and frequency of intercourse plays a vital role in increasing the chances of conception.

Subfertility: This means men may have a reduced ability to conceive but are not infertile.

1.4 The Women's Reproductive Health

Women's reproductive health refers to a wide range of elements pertaining to the female reproductive system such as the hormonal, psychological and physical elements that affect a woman's capacity to become pregnant, carry a healthy pregnancy until the end and deal with other obstacles to reproductive health. The essential elements of women's reproductive health are summarized as follows:

Menstrual Health: The menstrual cycle is a vital component of women's reproductive health. Assessing overall reproductive health requires an understanding of the menstrual cycle, tracking of periods, and recognition of irregularities.

Fertility: The ability of a woman to become pregnant and bring a child to life is referred to as fertility. Age, hormonal balance, and the existence of underlying medical conditions are some of the factors that influence fertility.

Conception and Pregnancy: Being capable to maintain an ideal pregnancy and the process of conception are both greatly influenced by reproductive health. To establish a healthy pregnancy, women must be aware of the elements that go into a successful conception and continue to receive the recommended prenatal care.

Hormonal Balance: The menstrual cycle and fertility are governed by hormones. Polycystic ovary syndrome (PCOS), irregular periods and problems with fertility can all be caused by disorders or imbalances in the production of hormones.

Menopause and Perimenopause: Menopause, or the actual transition from a woman's reproductive years to the menopause, is the end of a woman's reproductive years. One of the most important aspects of reproductive health is managing the mental and physical changes that come with these life stages.

Sexual Health: Preserving one's sexual health is vital for the general health and wellbeing of one's reproductive system. This includes treating problems like sexual dysfunction or pain.

Contraception: In order for women to make educated decisions about family planning, they must have access to information about the various forms of contraception. It's critical to comprehend the various forms of contraception and any possible side effects.

Reproductive Disorders and Conditions: A woman's ability to reproduce may be impacted by disorders like PCOS, uterine fibroids, and endometriosis. It's crucial to comprehend these illnesses and get the right medical attention.

Preventive Health: Early detection and prevention of reproductive and breast health issues, including cancer, depend on routine gynecological exams, Pap smears, and breast health screenings.

Mental and Emotional Health: Women's reproductive health is strongly correlated with their mental and emotional health. Emotional support and mental health treatment may be necessary when coping with problems like infertility or pregnancy loss.

Pelvic Health: Reproductive health depends on preserving a healthy pelvic floor. Sexual health and quality of life can be negatively impacted by pelvic floor disorders like prolapse and incontinence.

Access to Healthcare: A vital aspect of women's reproductive health is having access to high-quality reproductive healthcare, which includes family planning, prenatal care, and infertility treatment.

Education and Empowerment: Women are empowered to make decisions about their health and family planning when they are informed about their bodies, reproductive health, and available options.

Chapter 2: Assessing Your Fertility

2.1 Signs and Symptoms of Fertility Issues

Both men and women can have fertility problems. In about 20% of infertile couples, both partners have fertility problems. In about 15% of couples, no cause is found after all tests have been done. This is called unexplained infertility.

The main symptom of infertility is not getting pregnant. You may not have or notice any other symptoms. Symptoms can also depend on what is causing the infertility. Many health conditions can make it hard to get pregnant. Sometimes no cause is found.

In women, changes in the menstrual cycle and ovulation may be a symptom of a disease related to infertility. Symptoms include:

- Abnormal periods: Bleeding is heavier or lighter than usual.
- Irregular periods: The number of days in between each period varies each month.
- No periods: You have never had a period, or periods suddenly stop.
- Painful periods: Back pain, pelvic pain, and cramping may happen.

Sometimes, female infertility is related to a hormone problem. In this case, symptoms can also include:

- Skin changes, including more acne
- Changes in sex drive and desire

- Dark hair growth on the lips, chest, and chin
- Loss of hair or thinning hair
- Weight gain

Other symptoms of disorders that may lead to infertility include:

- Milky white discharge from nipples unrelated to breastfeeding
- Pain during sex

Many other things can be related to infertility in women, and their symptoms vary.

Infertility symptoms in men can be vague. They may go unnoticed until a man tries to have a baby. Symptoms depend on what is causing the infertility. They can include:

- Changes in hair growth

- Changes in sexual desire

- Pain, lump, or swelling in the testicles

- Problems with erections and ejaculation

- Small, firm testicles

2.2 Emotional Impact of Fertility Challenges

For a woman that has yearned for a baby for years, coming to terms with infertility problems can be devastating. The pressure one puts on oneself is bad enough but imagine the constant questioning by family and friends about when they are going to start a family. Over the years, a woman is inundated by expectations of motherhood through family members, films, media, and even self-talk. Not being able to conceive or having a partner with an infertility diagnosis can stir feelings of failure or inadequacy.

Just as a woman can be deeply affected by infertility, the male partner can experience similar mental anguish. Studies show depression, low self-esteem, and sexual dysfunction are common among men dealing with infertility. Some men may not express their feelings to their own partner, let alone their friends. Many have been raised to suppress their feelings, so experiencing such deep emotions may cause confusion, anger, and frustration. With males, they may yearn to be a father but are not socially pressured as women are with constant questioning by their peers. It can be more of a personal feeling of disappointment than embarrassment.

It's hard to know how to describe the emotional suffering couples face during fertility challenges. Couples have to try to come to terms with their own issues while seeing their friends and colleagues beginning their future with pregnancies. Life continues for the world while one's world seems to crumble.

As with any obstacle within a relationship, fertility problems can either make or break a couple. The grief and unknown of an infertility issue may cause a couple to turn to each other for support or cause marital distress.

2.3 Seeking Professional Help

There are a variety of reasons for seeking out a therapist to work through infertility challenges. It may be that your reproductive endocrinologist recommends or requires you to see a counselor before certain treatments, like when deciding to use a sperm or egg donor. Egg and sperm donors themselves are required to see a mental health counselor before they are allowed to donate.

For LGBTQ couples, counseling can help you consider your options for building a family and how different choices might affect your relationship. While you may not be facing a medical diagnosis of infertility, a counselor can help you with the process of assisted reproduction or adoption.

The emotional pain women experience when going through infertility can be severe and traumatic. (A research study from 1993 found that women with infertility experienced anxiety and depression at rates similar to those with cancer, heart conditions, and high blood pressure). Coping with infertility is difficult and needing help is 100 percent normal. Seeing a therapist could help you cope with the emotional struggle of infertility.

Chapter 3: Fertility Testing and Diagnosis

3.1 Fertility Medications and Hormone Therapy

If you've been unable to conceive within a reasonable period of time, seek help from your doctor for evaluation and treatment of infertility. You and your partner should be evaluated. Your doctor will take a detailed medical history and conduct a physical exam.

Fertility tests might include:

Ovulation Testing: An at-home, over-the-counter ovulation prediction kit detects the surge in luteinizing hormone (LH) that occurs before ovulation. A blood test for progesterone — a hormone produced after ovulation — can also document that you're ovulating. Other hormone levels, such as prolactin, also might be checked.

Hysterosalpingography:During hysterosalpingography (his-tur-o-sal-ping-GOG-ruh-fee), X-ray contrast is injected into your uterus and an X-ray is taken to check for problems inside the uterus. The test also shows whether the fluid passes out of the uterus and spills out of your fallopian tubes. If any problems are found, you'll likely need further evaluation.

Ovarian Reserve Testing: This testing helps determine the quality and quantity of eggs available for ovulation. Women at risk of a depleted egg supply — including women older than 35 — might have this series of blood and imaging tests.

Other Hormone Testing: Other hormone tests check levels of ovulatory hormones as well as thyroid and pituitary hormones that control reproductive processes.

Imaging Tests: A pelvic ultrasound looks for uterine or fallopian tube disease. Sometimes a sonohysterogram, also called a saline infusion sonogram, or a hysteroscopy is used to see details inside the uterus that can't be seen on a regular ultrasound.

Depending on your situation, rarely your testing might include:
Laparoscopy: This minimally invasive surgery involves making a small incision beneath your navel and inserting a thin viewing device to examine your fallopian tubes, ovaries and uterus.

A laparoscopy can identify endometriosis, scarring, blockages or irregularities of the fallopian tubes, and problems with the ovaries and uterus.

Genetic Testing: Genetic testing helps determine whether there are any changes to your genes that may be causing infertility.

Fertility Medications

Infertility treatment depends on the cause, your age, how long you've been infertile and personal preferences. Because infertility is a complex disorder, treatment involves significant financial, physical, psychological and time commitments. Treatments can either attempt to restore fertility through medication or surgery, or help you get pregnant with sophisticated techniques. Medications that regulate or stimulate ovulation are known as fertility drugs. Fertility drugs are the main treatment for women who are infertile due to ovulation disorders.

Fertility drugs generally work like natural hormones — follicle-stimulating hormone (FSH) and luteinizing hormone (LH) — to trigger ovulation. They're also used in women who ovulate to try to stimulate a better egg or an extra egg or eggs.

Fertility drugs include:
Clomiphene Citrate: Taken by mouth, this drug stimulates ovulation by causing the pituitary gland to release more follicle-stimulating hormone (FSH) and luteinizing hormone (LH), which stimulate the growth of an ovarian follicle containing an egg. This is generally the first line

treatment for women younger than 39 who don't have polycystic ovary syndrome (PCOS).

Gonadotropins: These injected treatments stimulate the ovary to produce multiple eggs. Gonadotropin medications include human menopausal gonadotropin or hMG (Menopur) and FSH (Gonal-F, Follistim AQ, Bravelle). Another gonadotropin, human chorionic gonadotropin (Ovidrel, Pregnyl), is used to mature the eggs and trigger their release at the time of ovulation. Concerns exist that there's a higher risk of conceiving multiples and having a premature delivery with gonadotropin use.

Metformin: This drug is used when insulin resistance is a known or suspected cause of infertility, usually in women with a diagnosis of PCOS. Metformin (Fortamet) helps improve insulin resistance, which can improve the likelihood of ovulation.

Letrozole: Letrozole (Femara) belongs to a class of drugs known as aromatase inhibitors and works in a similar fashion to clomiphene. Letrozole is usually used for woman younger than 39 who have PCOS.

Bromocriptine: Bromocriptine (Cycloset, Parlodel), a dopamine agonist, might be used when ovulation problems are caused by excess production of prolactin (hyperprolactinemia) by the pituitary gland.

For couples struggling to conceive, hormonal therapy can be a life-changing solution as many cases of infertility can be attributed to hormonal imbalances. Hormone treatments work by controlled ovarian hyperstimulation to promote egg maturation and ovulation. The hormones are usually injected either beneath the skin or into the muscle. The site of injection could be your upper arm, upper thigh, buttocks, or stomach. They are administered for 7 to 12 consecutive days with the first injection given on the 2nd or 3rd day after you notice bright red blood from your menstrual period. You may need to take them along with clomiphene citrate (Clomid), which is an estrogen-blocking drug that causes release of hormones that stimulate egg production

Here's a list of 5 hormone treatments for infertility:

Gonadotropin: Releasing Hormone Agonist (GnRH agonist): Brand names are Lupron, Synarel, and Zoladex. They may be administered as injections or nasal sprays and function by preventing premature ovulation during in vitro fertilization (IVF), gamete intrafallopian transfer (GIFT) or other assisted reproductive technology (ART) retrieval cycles.

Human Menopausal Gonadotropins (hMG): Brand names include Pergonal, Humegon, and Repronex. They are administered as intramuscular or subcutaneous injections. They stimulate ovaries during ART procedures.

Follicle-Stimulating Hormone (FSH): Brand names are Follistim, Gonal F, and Fertinex. They are administered as subcutaneous injections and are generally prescribed for patients not responding to Clomid or as part of ART treatment.

Human Chorionic Gonadotropin (hCG): Brand names include Novarel and Pregnyl. They are administered as intramuscular injections and usually used in combination with other fertility medication to induce timed ovulation.

Progesterone: It may be administered as an intramuscular injection. This hormone supports development of your uterine lining and prepares it for embryo implantation. Progesterone supplementation is often used in combination with GnRH agonists in treating infertility.

Due to the non-invasive nature of hormone treatments, they may be used at a very early stage once hormonal imbalances are identified; however, hormone treatments can cause side effects such as bloating, mood swings, irritability, increased cravings, and blood clots.

To maximize positive outcomes and reduce risk of side effects, it is best that hormone treatments are administered by certified reproductive specialists.

3.2 Assisted Reproductive Technology

ART refers to medical procedures that aim to achieve pregnancy. These complex treatments involve influencing gametes, or eggs and sperm, to increase the chances of fertilization. ART is typically an option for people for whom other infertility treatments may not work or those who have already tried treatment but have not become pregnant.

People considering ART will often discuss options with a healthcare professional and may require a consultation from a fertility specialist. While people primarily use ART to address infertility, others may use it for genetic purposes or avoid pregnancy complications. Some people may also refer to ART as fertility treatment or medically assisted reproduction. It may be difficult for many people to access fertility services such as ART due to its high cost and limited coverage by private insurance and Medicaid.

3.3 In Vitro Fertilization

IVF involves a doctor extracting eggs and fertilizing them in a special lab. Specialists can combine this with an embryo transfer (IVF-ET) and transfer the resulting embryos into a person's uterus. The Society for Assisted Reproductive Technology states that IVF-ET accounts for 99% of ART procedures.

The Centers for Disease Control and Prevention (CDC) lists the 2018 success rates of IVF treatments for one oocyte retrieval from people using their own eggs as:

- 52% for people aged 35 or younger
- 38.1% for people aged 35–37
- 23.5% for people aged 38–40
- 7.6% for those over the age of 40

A person may also use a tool called an IVF success estimator to estimate their chance of having a baby using IVF.

It may take more than one IVF cycle to result in pregnancy and some people may not conceive with IVF at all. The benefits of IVF are an increased chance of fertilization and pregnancy. Potential complications may include:

- multiple pregnancy, or two or more embryos implanting at a time

- side effects from fertility drugs, such as ovarian hyperstimulation syndrome
- ectopic pregnancy, where the embryo settles outside of the womb

3.4 Egg Donation and Surrogacy

Egg donation is a process in which a fertile woman donates an egg or oocyte to another woman to help her conceive. It is a part of assisted reproductive technology (ART). The procedure typically involves a doctor removing an egg or eggs from the donor, fertilizing them in a laboratory, and then transferring the resulting embryos into the recipient's uterus. Doctors do this using an implantation procedure, such as in vitro fertilization (IVF). Sometimes, specialists at the facility may freeze some or all of the embryos for later use or implantation in different women. Egg donation frequently benefits women who cannot use their own eggs for various reasons, including ovarian failure, avoiding congenital anomalies in the fetus, or advanced age.

In this subsection, we'll look at the criteria for selecting donors, the procedure itself and legal ramifications following an egg donation.

What To Expect

Specialists at the fertility facility will conduct an intensive selection process to find a suitable donor and will carefully run through the legal procedures. Before starting the procedure, most donors will need to take medication that stops their normal menstrual cycle.

Side effects of this medication might include:
- hot flashes

- headache

- fatigue

- body aches

The donor will then take a series of fertility drugs that stimulate the ovaries to produce several eggs at once. This is known as hyperstimulation. Donors will need to self-administer this medication by injecting it under their skin or into a muscle. Some women may experience mild side effects, such as bruising at the injection site, mood swings, and tender breasts. In rare cases, a woman may develop severe ovarian hyperstimulation syndrome (OHSS). This occurs when too many eggs develop in the ovaries. Women who develop OHSS may require hospitalization. Donors do have a risk of pregnancy before the eggs are retrieved, so it is a good idea to avoid intercourse or use a barrier contraceptive, such as a condom.

Throughout the donation cycle, a donor will undergo frequent blood tests and ultrasound examinations to monitor their reactions to the medications.

During Extraction

Shortly before the retrieval of the eggs, the donor will receive a final injection in preparation for the procedure. The doctor will perform a transvaginal ovarian aspiration to remove the eggs from the donor's ovaries. They will insert an ultrasound probe into the vagina and use a needle to remove the egg from each follicle. During the procedure, which lasts around 30 minutes, the doctor might give the donor painkillers, sedatives, or an anesthetic. As this is a minor procedure, a donor will not need to stay at the clinic or hospital overnight.

After Donation

Some women find they need several days of rest to recover from the transvaginal ovarian aspiration. Others return to normal activities the next day. Some programs provide aftercare to donors but others do not. As the egg donation process can have a psychological impact, some women may find it useful to work with a counselor or psychotherapist after the procedure.

Let's have a look at surrogacy. Surrogacy is an arrangement, often supported by a legal agreement, whereby a woman agrees to deliver/labor on behalf of another couple or person, who will become the child's parent(s) after birth. People may seek a surrogacy arrangement when a couple do not wish to carry a pregnancy themselves, when pregnancy is medically impossible, when pregnancy risks are dangerous for the intended mother, or when a single man or a male same sex couple wish to have a child. In surrogacy arrangements, monetary compensation may or may not be involved. Receiving money for the arrangement is known as commercial surrogacy. The legality and cost of surrogacy varies widely between jurisdictions, sometimes resulting in problematic international or interstate surrogacy arrangements. Couples seeking a surrogacy arrangement in a country where it is banned sometimes travel to a jurisdiction that permits it. In some countries, surrogacy is legal only if money is not exchanged. Where commercial surrogacy is legal, couples may use the help of third-party agencies to assist in the process of surrogacy by finding a surrogate and arranging a surrogacy contract with her. These agencies often screen surrogates' psychological and other medical tests to ensure the best chance of healthy gestation and delivery. They also usually facilitate all legal matters concerning the intended parents and the surrogate.

3.5 Adoption as an Alternative

Adoption is one of a range of alternatives that you may be considering if you cannot conceive and give birth to a child. You may have experienced miscarriages or secondary infertility. The following information will be particularly relevant if you are exploring adoption due to fertility issues or you are thinking of taking the next step.

There is no upper age limit for adoption, unlike assisted conception, so don't feel that you have to rush if you have tried fertility treatments without success. The adoption process nowadays is much faster than it used to be, and you could be approved to adopt in as little as six months. It is advisable to take a break after your last treatment or after a miscarriage, and adoption agencies will often prefer that you wait at least 6 months before starting an adoption assessment.

Adoption is a great way to become a parent but not a direct alternative to conception. It is important to take time to work through grieving and loss to feel emotionally ready to move on and devote your energies to adoption. If you are a couple you both need to feel ready for the adoption process.

You don't have to try fertility treatments first. Adoption can be a positive first choice if you are unable to conceive. Some people have moral or religious objections to assisted conception, some would rather avoid any unpleasant symptoms and side effects of treatment, some consider the prospects of success too slim, and some find their motivation to love and parent a child or children that need a family is stronger than the biological drive to produce a child that shares their genes.

You have the strength to become an adopter. If you have undergone fertility treatment and are now considering adoption, you have already been through a lot. Research shows that for many couples coping with infertility strengthens their relationship. Adoption agencies welcome couples whose relationships are resilient and have stood the test of time, and you may have learned a lot about dealing with stress and emotional challenges which will stand you in good stead when you become a parent.

Already have children? Consider their needs. If you have secondary infertility (unable to have a second or subsequent child) adoption can be a great way to increase or complete your family. How to prepare for this and the needs of your existing child or children will be an important part of the assessment. Agencies will generally want the adopted child to be the youngest in the family by at least 2 years and preferably more, as a reasonable age gap and giving each child space has been shown in research to be beneficial.

You are unlikely to adopt a baby. It is common for potential adopters who have fertility issues to want to adopt a baby as young as possible. It is alright to be honest about this if it is part of your motivation to adopt, but it also helps if you have a realistic idea of the children who need adoptive families. Most children adopted are between 12 months to 4 years old, and it is rare for a baby to be voluntarily relinquished at birth. All adopted children will need lots of love, nurture, time and attention from their new parent(s). Ask adoption agencies about the age range of children they are looking for parents for and consider keeping an open mind, as many adopters find their views change during the assessment process.

Agencies will be sensitive to your situation. All adoption agencies are likely to have experience of assessing people who are considering adoption due to infertility or difficulties conceiving. You can expect agencies to deal sensitively with your enquiries. When you are starting the adoption process with an adoption agency they will ask about your motivation to adopt and will also ask that you don't attempt to conceive once you are being assessed to adopt.

If you feel ready to approach an adoption agency you can search for local agencies and chat things through with a few as they are happy to give information and answer questions even if you're not yet sure about adoption, so do contact them if you want to find out more.

Chapter 4: Lifestyle Factors and Fertility

4.1 Nutrition and Diet for Fertility

If you're trying to conceive, changing your diet can prepare your body for pregnancy. We rounded up foods that increase fertility for optimal chances of conception—plus some items to eliminate from your meal plan. While there aren't any magic foods for getting pregnant, one simple way to support your fertility is ensuring your diet includes healthy choices from the following food groups.

Fruits and Vegetables: Load your plate with fruits and veggies. A study which comprised nearly 18,000 women, found a higher incidence of ovulatory disorder in those who consumed more trans fats, sugar from carbohydrates, and animal proteins. On the other hand, those who consumed more iron, fiber, and protein from vegetables had a higher fertility diet score. What does this mean for people trying to conceive? Make sure half your plate at every meal is composed of fresh fruits and vegetables.

Fats: Healthy, plant-based fats in moderation are an important part of any balanced diet. Nuts, avocados, olive oil, and grapeseed oil can reduce the inflammation in the body—and studies have shown that anti-inflammatory diets can lead to improved fertility. Some fats may even assist people who truly struggle with infertility.Studies have shown that consuming a certain quantity of monounsaturated fats during the IVF cycle increased the success rate by three and a half times, as opposed to women who don't eat good plant-based fats during that period. Foods high in monounsaturated fat include avocados, nuts, and some oils (like olive oil, peanut oil, and canola oil).

It can also be helpful to avoid trans fats (the kind found in processed snacks like French fries and packaged foods) and eat more unsaturated fats. Trans fats increase insulin resistance. Insulin helps move glucose from the bloodstream to the cells; resistance means it's harder to move glucose into the cells. The pancreas keeps pumping out more insulin anyway, resulting in more insulin in your bloodstream. High insulin levels can negatively affect ovulation, so it's best to focus on foods that guard against insulin resistance when creating a fertility diet.

Complex Carbs: To increase fertility, try to incorporate more complex ("slow") carbs and limit highly processed ones. Your body digests refined carbs (like cookies, cakes, white bread, and white rice) quickly, and turns them into blood sugar. To drive down the blood-sugar spike, the pancreas releases insulin into the bloodstream, and studies have found that high insulin levels appear to inhibit ovulation. Complex carbs (those containing fiber, such as fruits, vegetables, beans, and whole grains) are digested slowly and have a more gradual effect on blood sugar and insulin. Barely refined grains are also superb sources of fertility-friendly B vitamins, vitamin E, and fiber.

Protein: Chicken, turkey, pork, and beef trimmed of excess fat are great sources of protein, zinc, and iron—all-important building blocks for a healthy pregnancy. Excess saturated fat found in animal protein, on the other hand, may be linked to fertility issues, according to one study on nutrition and fertility. Protein sources from the sea can also be nutritious options. For instance, coldwater fish like salmon, canned light tuna, and sardines are excellent sources of DHA and omega-3 fatty acids; they also help develop the baby's nervous system and cut your risk of premature birth, so why not start pre-conception?

You can include these fish options a couple of times a week in a fertility diet without worrying about mercury levels. But it's best to avoid other varieties, such as shark, swordfish, tilefish, and king mackerel, which are known for having higher levels of mercury. Eggs, too, are another potent protein source in a fertility diet. They get a bad rap from cholesterol, but the yolk has excellent stores of protein and choline, a vitamin that helps develop brain function in babies.

Dairy: Lactose-tolerant people should reach for whole milk or other full-fat dairy foods (such as yogurt) instead of non-fat and low-fat dairy to support fertility. The more low-fat dairy products in a woman's diet, the more trouble she had getting pregnant. That's because a high intake of low-fat dairy has been shown to raise the risk of ovulatory infertility compared to high-fat dairy.

Foods to Limit or Avoid in a Fertility Diet
Everyone's fertility diet will look different, and it's important to always listen to your body when it comes to nutrition. But if you're looking specifically to get pregnant, it may be helpful to know how the following foods can impact your

fertility. This way, your food choices can come from a place of empowerment.

Caffeine: If you're a java lover, you don't have to completely eliminate your daily brew, but it may be helpful to consume coffee and tea in moderation when trying to get pregnant. Consumption of coffee or tea doesn't seem to cause ovulation problems but it could lead to dehydration. In addition, caffeine is a diuretic that can prevent your mucus membranes from staying moist, potentially affecting the consistency of your cervical mucus. (The more fertile cervical mucus you have, the better chances the sperm has of "sticking" to it and reaching the egg.)

Instead, consider replacing some of your daily caffeine with decaffeinated or low-caf beverages, decaf coffee, and herbal teas.

Alcohol: Most experts recommend that couples looking to get pregnant avoid alcohol. Not only can it lead to dehydration, but high amounts of alcohol use (this includes binge drinking) have been associated with reduced fertility. Additionally, if you're regularly drinking and get pregnant without realizing it, there may be some risks to the fetus as well. It's also important to note that the benefits of abstaining don't just apply to the person getting pregnant but also to the man as alcohol use can impair sperm health and may have lasting effects on the fetus too.

Bottom line? If you're looking to get pregnant, it might be best for you and your partner to limit alcohol for now.

Sugary Drinks and Processed Sweeteners: It's important to live a balanced life with treats now and then. But if you have any issues with unstable blood sugar levels (for instance, if you have diabetes or PCOS), it might be helpful to stick to less-processed sweeteners to help boost fertility. Concentrated doses of the sweet stuff can throw your blood sugar totally out of whack, creating issues with insulin and your general hormonal balance. Consume candies and desserts in moderation for your fertility diet plan, and don't forget about sneakier sugar bombs like fruit juice, energy drinks, and sweet teas. Sugared sodas, in particular, have been associated with ovulatory infertility.

Processed Soy: It may be helpful to avoid forms of processed soy in your fertility diet, particularly powders and energy bars, because research suggests that soy may have a negative effect on fertility.

4.2 Exercise and Stress Management

One of the most debated subjects revolving around the ability to become pregnant is exercise. While you may feel tremendously fragile at this time, we can assure you exercise won't harm you. In fact, the right amount of exercise, and the type of exercise you perform, may actually enhance your fertility and improve your quest to conceive. Keeping active while trying to become pregnant helps you in so many ways. Regular aerobic exercise, those activities that increase your heart rate and get your blood pumping is essential to a healthy cardiovascular system. When you work out you increase your endorphins which help alleviate stress and who isn't experiencing a little stress when trying to conceive? Although exercise is recommended for many women, before and during pregnancy, there are a few caveats. If there is any reason why you shouldn't perform even low-impact exercise, consult your physician. Always let your doctor know what kind of workouts you favor most, how often and how vigorously you work out.

The Best Kinds of Exercise for Your Fertility
Moderate forms of exercise for five hours or less per week are typically recommended for healthy women of all body types. If you usually go hard and heavy in your workout endeavors, try scaling back on intensity. Replace your strenuous exercise with one of these recommended workouts:

Walking: Walking is always a safe way to get your exercise. It's excellent for your cardiovascular system, builds endurance, is low-impact, and a great stress-buster.

Dancing: Dancing helps you bust a move and improve blood flow. Dancing also offers a decent calorie-burn.

Bicycling: Bicycling for 30 minutes few times a week is a wonderful way to get your workout in. Just make sure you're safe; wear a helmet and watch out for careless drivers if you're sharing the road.

Yoga: Yoga can be a phenomenal way to limber up (great for delivering a baby!) and relax. A yoga body is strong and sleek, and yoga can definitely help you deal with the stress of infertility. Whether you practice yoga at home, or work out in a studio, don't push your body too far.

Pilates: Pilates is another beneficial way to stay healthy and improve your fertility. Pilates is relaxing, while still offering a challenge.

Swimming: Swimming for exercise is one if the best ways to work out. You can get a thorough cardio workout without putting too much stress on your joints. Swimming for fitness allows you to set the pace that's most comfortable and build on it. This is an excellent choice for those just starting a fitness routine.

Always listen to your body, and stay hydrated. You never want to put yourself at risk for a fall, or injury, and remember you could become pregnant at any time, so go easy if you aren't into regular exercise.

Now let's have a good look at stress management. "Stress" refers to the response of the sympathetic nervous system to a triggering event. The body releases hormones, such as adrenaline, into the bloodstream, resulting in the "fight or flight" reaction. This physiological response helps us become more alert, motivated, and ready to respond to real or perceived danger. Have you ever felt your heart race or your breath quicken? How about when your face gets flushed or your hands get sweaty? This is part of your body's normal and healthy response to stress.

However, stress can have a negative effect on your body if it becomes continuous or chronic. In the short term, chronic stress can lead you to have difficulties falling asleep, causing you to toss and turn all night. We've all been there, right? It can cause you to eat poorly, increase substance use, and/or become irritable. Long-term stress can lead to increased blood pressure, upset stomach, headaches, and can also lower immune system functioning. From a psychological standpoint, chronic stress can eventually result in depression, panic attacks, and anxiety. Stress is a part of most fertility journeys, but thankfully, there are things you can do to combat some of this natural response in a healthy way.

Make a List of Priorities: Before taking on new commitments, evaluate whether now is the right time to add something else to your plate. Don't be afraid to say no to requests from friends, family or work to ensure you don't get overwhelmed.

Find a Fertility Friend or Support Group: Support groups are a safe place to vent, talk about how you're really doing, and hear from others who can relate. Social media platforms also have strong fertility communities and can help you find new friends by connecting you to others who truly understand what you're going through.

Get to Know Yourself Again: What are some things you enjoy doing? What are your hobbies? Who's in your support network? How have you handled stress in the past? There is no one-size-fits-all way to deal with stress, but learning about yourself will help you hatch a personalized self-care plan that works for you.

Remember, It's Okay to Take Breaks: Taking some time to reconnect with your interests and life outside of fertility treatment can be incredibly restorative. Explore things you once enjoyed that may have taken a backseat due to treatment, like painting, crafting, volunteering, or other activities!

Practice Breath Work: Find some breathing exercises that feel good to you (for example, box breathing) or utilize a relaxation or mindfulness app for some guided breathwork.

Trust Your Care Team: Remember to rely on your physician and Care Team for medical advice instead of advice from unqualified people. Your team will be able to provide tailored advice and support and answer any questions or concerns you may have.

Seek Out a Therapist: A good therapist can provide you with professional guidance as you manage infertility and fertility treatment.

Create a Mental Health Toolbox: Building a mental health toolbox is an incredibly helpful way to ensure your self-care resources are close at hand for difficult days. You can do this by creating a list on your phone, putting items (like a stress ball or favorite candle) in a physical box, or whatever works best for you. Here are some suggestions for what to add to your toolbox: photos of loved ones, encouraging notes from friends or family, positive affirmations, meditation or relaxation apps, a playlist of your favorite songs to cheer you on, phone numbers of people you trust, or other tools.

Recognize Infertility as a Life Crisis: The emotional and physical impact of infertility and fertility treatment should not be understated. Acknowledging the sadness, disappointment, and stress associated with infertility is an important step in the process. Infertility is a big deal, and there is nothing "wrong" with you if you're struggling to accept or navigate it. By recognizing the true impact of infertility, you allow yourself the space to process it and be gentle with yourself.

4.3 Holistic Approaches to Fertility

Medicine isn't a straightforward concept. There are typically multiple approaches to treatment for any number of conditions and fertility is no different. The options below are holistic approach in addressing fertility:

Acupuncture: Acupuncture is a traditional Chinese medicine treatment that has been around for ages. The process involves placing painless, thin needles strategically within the body in a grid-like pattern. The needles stimulate energy points within the body that are believed to regulate wellness in the body. These points promote mental, physical, emotional, and spiritual balance. This allows the body to unwind and relax so that the mind and body can focus on fertility. A study in 2002 found that the addition of acupuncture treatments to traditional in vitro fertilization treatment dramatically increased the results of a successful pregnancy.

Mind Body Medicine: When the body is not in a healthy state of being, fertility can become difficult. Depression, anxiety, anger, insomnia, fatigue, and isolation can all contribute to this difficulty and decrease the chance of conception. By utilizing an approach that focuses on improving the mental state along with the physical state, patients increase their chances of conception at least three-fold.

Chapter 5: Coping With Fertility Stress

5.1 Communicating With a Supportive Community

Infertility can be a difficult and isolating experience, but connecting with others who understand what you're going through can be incredibly helpful. Joining a supportive community, whether online or in person, can provide you with the validation, understanding, and resources you need to feel less alone. Here are some tips for communicating with a supportive community:

Finding a Community that Shares Your Values and Goals: There are many online communities for people who are experiencing infertility, including message boards, forums, and social media groups. You can also find in-person support groups through organizations like local hospitals. When looking for a supportive community, try to find one that aligns with your values and goals. For example, some groups focus on emotional support, while others focus on specific treatment options or advocacy.

Respecting Other Members' Privacy and Confidentiality: In any supportive community, it's important to respect the privacy and confidentiality of other members. This means not sharing personal information about other members without their permission. It also means being mindful of the sensitive nature of the topic. Avoid making assumptions or judgments about other members, and always approach the community with compassion and empathy.

Being Open and Honest About Your Own Experiences: When you're part of a supportive community, it's important to be open and honest about your own experiences. This can help you connect with others who have had similar experiences, and it can also help you feel less alone. It's okay to be vulnerable and share your struggles, and it can be cathartic to know that others understand what you're going through. However, it's also important to maintain healthy boundaries and not share more than you're comfortable with.

Offering Support and Encouragement to Others: In addition to receiving support from others, it's important to give support to other members of the community. This can be as simple as offering an encouraging word or listening to someone else's story. You can also offer advice or resources based on your own experiences. By giving support, you're helping to build a stronger and more supportive community.

Seeking Professional Help When Needed: While a supportive community can be incredibly helpful, it's important to remember that it's not a substitute for professional help. If you're struggling with your mental health, or if you're having difficulty coping with infertility, it's important to seek out professional help. A therapist or counselor can provide you with the tools and resources you need to manage your mental health. They can also help you develop healthy coping strategies for dealing with infertility.

5.2 Maintaining Strong Relationships

Infertility can be one of the biggest reasons why couples are not able to sustain their relationship. Many times, the partner in whom some fertility issue is diagnosed may suffer from discrimination and blame by the other partner. This can cause a lot of guilt, shame and mental agony in the infertile partner. These intimate tensions can slowly percolate in daily life circumstances and lead to a strained relationship. So, how do you nourish a healthy relationship as you combat infertility problems? Here's how you should nurture a healthy relationship while tackling infertility issues.

Don't Shame Your Partner: Both partners should understand that the diagnosis of infertility is equally stressful for each other. In addition, the partner with fertility problem suffers with unwanted guilt and shame. This is the time when one needs the support of their partner the most. Be vocal about your problems. If you are not at the receiving end of the problem, you should not feel shameful or look down upon your partner. Avoid bringing the topic of fertility and its problems while arguing on some other unrelated matter.

Address Each Other's Fears: One of the most common fears couples avoid addressing is the fear of one's partner leaving them if they are the ones with the infertility problem. Many women harbor a deep-seated fear of being abandoned by their partner for someone much younger. It is always better to address one's fear early on in their fertility journey than later. If not addressed, then the partner suffers from self-blame, low self-esteem and infertility stress, which can hamper the relationship.

Avoid Resentment and Misunderstanding: It is humane to feel sad and low when we do not get what we desire. At the same time, every individual has their own way to cope with stress. Some like to talk about how they are feeling, some like to keep it low. Many times, women feel unloved and have strong resentment against their partners for not caring enough!! Onc must understand that each one has their own way of coping with stress. Avoid misunderstandings and agree to differ in your opinions and the way both partners react to the same emotional stress. That helps in nourishing one's relationship in one's fertility journey.

Communicate and Seek Help When Required: Communication is key to a healthy relationship. Talk to each other and convey your feelings. At the same time, one must know that talking everyday about the same fertility problem can be depressing. So, keeping a balance is important. Share your emotions and convey fears but not all the time. Reassure each other. Keep the conversation short and light. Seek the help of your health professionals who can help you clear your doubts. At times talking to your close friends and family members can also help. Don't carry the burden and stress all by yourself.

Try to Laugh More: No matter how stressful it looks, it is always nice to add fun and humor in your relationship. It lightens the burden. Laughing together releases "happy hormones" which not only makes you feel better, it is actually a stress buster. Always remember this is just a phase, it will get over soon. Remember what doesn't break you, make you. Be hopeful and be kind to each other. Support one another and see your relationship blossom even in the toughest phases of your life.

Chapter 6: Pregnancy and Beyond

6.1 Preconception and Prenatal Care

Preconception care consists of the healthcare you receive before conceiving. During this time, your doctor will assess your health to determine if there are conditions that can affect your future pregnancy. Potential risks may be reduced or eliminated by applying interventions such as medication or lifestyle changes. Lifestyle changes that are encouraged may include eating a healthy diet, maintaining a healthy weight, taking supplements that contain folic acid, receiving pertinent vaccinations, getting mentally healthy, quitting smoking and avoiding alcohol consumption.

There are many benefits associated with preconception care, they include:

- Reducing infant and maternal mortality
- Reducing the risk of complications during pregnancy
- Preventing certain birth defects

Most doctors recommend receiving preconception care three to six months before the time you intend to conceive.

Prenatal care is healthcare you receive while you are pregnant. It is important because it helps improve your chances of having a healthy pregnancy. Your visits with your doctor may involve physical exams, imaging tests, blood tests or screening tests to detect fetal abnormalities. It is recommended that you ask your physician lots of questions and express your concerns during these visits. Your physician will serve as a guide and source of support as your body changes.

Women who receive regular prenatal care may receive benefits that include:

- Reducing the risk of pregnancy complications
- Managing preexisting medical conditions such as high blood pressure which can affect pregnancy
- Receiving accurate nutritional information
- Ensuring that medications being taken are safe
- Physician monitoring of the baby's development
- Decreasing the possibility of preterm labor.

Prenatal care is essential in promoting the best possible outcomes for mother and child. The sooner you receive care the better.

6.2 Parenting After Infertility

In many ways, parenting after infertility is no different from general parenting. Your life brims with typical parenting concerns like getting your kids to sleep, trying new foods, and setting your child up for success in school. However, you are a different person and, therefore, a different kind of parent because you struggled with infertility. And your child, whether they've come to you through adoption, foster care, or third-party reproduction, has a few key differences that require extra attention and intention as you raise them.

It is worth thinking about some unique ways infertility might affect your parenting style. How did you handle your disappointment and grief? What did you learn about your strength and resilience? You likely navigated some challenging conversations and unwanted advice. All these struggles can inform how you parent a child who has felt their own loss and grief before joining your family. It's also valuable to consider how your child's history impacts their experience in your family. Learning about trauma, neglect, abuse, or prenatal substance exposure is not easy, but educating yourself about these topics will equip you to be the parent this child needs.

When raising a child through adoption, foster, kinship care, or a third-party reproductive process, you must also consider how and when

to tell them about their story in age-appropriate
and developmentally appropriate ways.

Conclusion: Your Fertility Journey Continues

As we reach the end of this guide, it's important to recognize that your fertility journey is an ongoing and dynamic process. This conclusion aims to offer encouragement, reflection, and a forward-looking perspective as you continue navigating the path towards parenthood.

Acknowledging Your Journey: Take a moment to acknowledge the steps you've already taken on your fertility journey. Whether you've explored medical treatments, considered alternative paths, or embarked on the adoption process, each decision reflects your commitment to building the family you envision.

Embracing Resilience: Fertility journeys often involve resilience in the face of challenges. Recognize the strength you've displayed, the lessons learned, and the personal growth experienced along the way. Your resilience is a testament to your determination and courage.

Seeking Support: Your journey doesn't have to be solitary. Consider reaching out to your support network—friends, family, or support groups—where you can share your experiences, receive encouragement, and connect with others who understand the complexities of the fertility journey.

Navigating Emotional Well-being: Emotional well-being is an integral part of any fertility journey. Whether you're celebrating successes, navigating uncertainties, or facing disappointments, prioritizing your mental and emotional health is key. Seek counseling, mindfulness practices, or other strategies that resonate with you.

Evaluating Options: Fertility paths are diverse, and your journey may involve exploring various options. Continuously assess what aligns with your values, priorities, and circumstances. Stay informed about advances in reproductive medicine, adoption processes, or any alternative approaches that may resonate with you.

Maintaining Open Communication: Communication, both with your partner and within your broader community, is crucial. Keep the lines of dialogue open, sharing your feelings, hopes, and concerns. A supportive network can provide valuable insights and perspectives, contributing to a sense of shared responsibility.

Cultivating Hope: Maintaining hope is a powerful force in any fertility journey. Embrace the possibilities that lie ahead, whether through continued medical treatments, adoption processes, or any other paths you choose. Cultivate a mindset that focuses on hope and the potential for positive outcomes.

Embracing Flexibility: Fertility journeys often unfold with unexpected twists and turns. Embrace flexibility in your plans, allowing room for adaptation and adjustments. Recognize that the journey itself may shape your goals and desires, leading to new possibilities.

Celebrating Milestones: Take time to celebrate the milestones, no matter how small, achieved along your fertility journey. Each step forward is a victory, and acknowledging these achievements can provide a sense of accomplishment and motivation.

Moving Forward with Confidence: As you continue your fertility journey, do so with confidence and a belief in your ability to navigate the challenges ahead. Trust in your resilience, the support around you, and your capacity to make informed decisions for your family-building goals.

If you're reading this book on fertility, you may also be interested in my book on breast cancer and prostate cancer. Tap the links above to read them.